TYPE 1 DIABETIC VEGETARIAN COOKBOOK

Delicious and Balanced Recipes for Type 1 Diabetics

By Mia Bennett

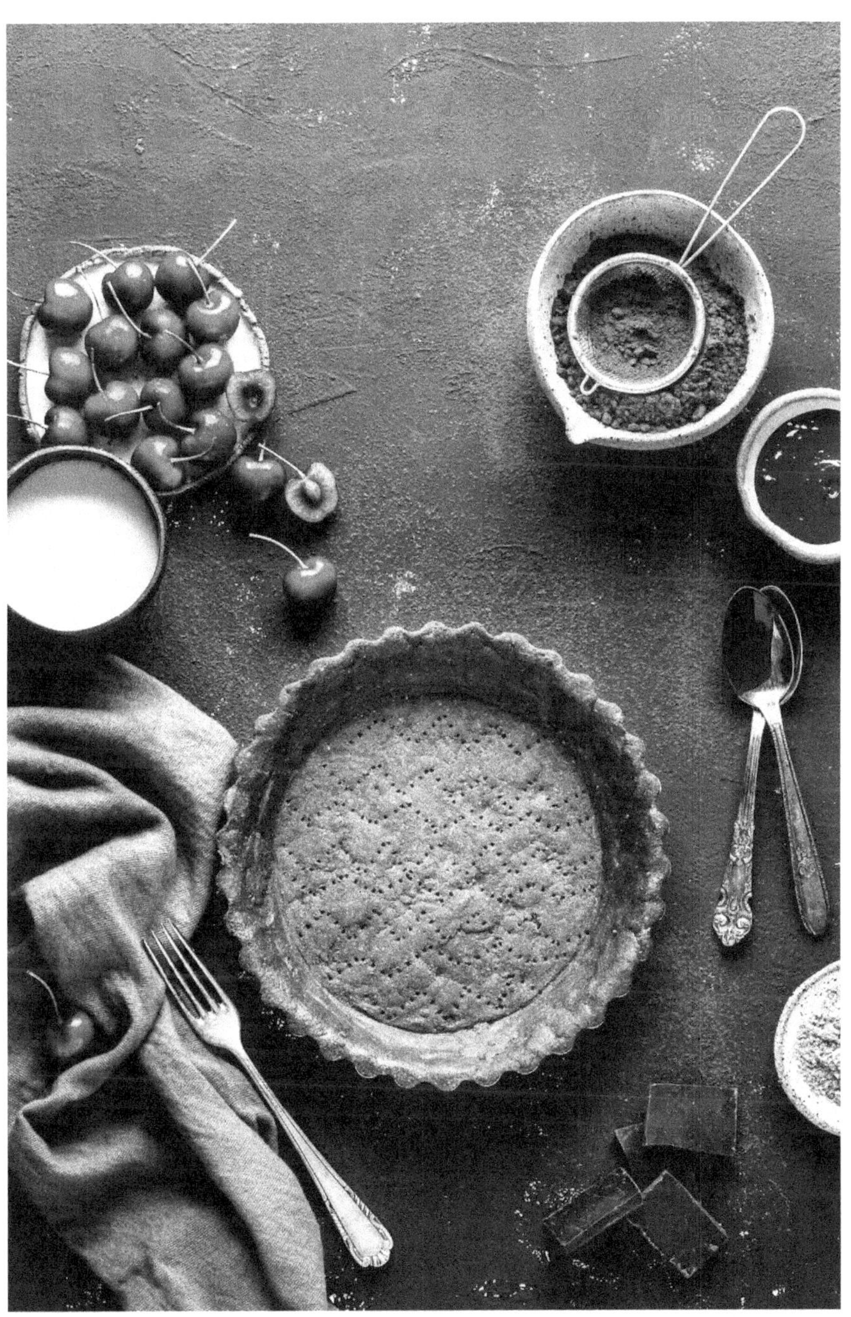

TABLE OF CONTENTS

INTRODUCTION

For those living with type 1 diabetes (T1D), managing blood sugar levels is a constant dance. This dance can take on a new dimension when considering a vegetarian lifestyle. While vegetarianism isn't a magic bullet for T1D, it can be a healthy and manageable approach with careful planning.

Understanding Type 1 Diabetes and Food

T1D is an autoimmune disease where the body attacks insulin-producing cells in the pancreas. Insulin is the key that unlocks cells, allowing them to absorb glucose (sugar) from the bloodstream for energy. Without enough insulin, blood sugar levels rise, leading to a cascade of health problems.

Food plays a central role in T1D management. Carbohydrates (carbs) are the main source of blood sugar, so understanding how different foods affect blood sugar levels is crucial. This is where vegetarianism comes in.

Benefits of a Vegetarian Diet for Type 1 Diabetics

- **Fiber Powerhouse**: Vegetarian diets are naturally rich in fiber, which slows down carbohydrate digestion, leading to steadier blood sugar levels.

- **Weight Management:** Vegetarian diets tend to be lower in calories and fat, which can aid in weight management. Maintaining a healthy weight can significantly improve blood sugar control.

- **Heart-Healthy Benefits:** Vegetarian diets are often linked to lower cholesterol and blood pressure, both of which are beneficial for overall health, especially for those with T1D who are at higher risk of heart disease.

Key Nutritional Considerations

- **Protein Planning:** With animal products off the menu, getting enough protein is essential. Plant-based protein sources like legumes (beans, lentils), tofu, tempeh, and nuts can be incorporated throughout the day.

- **Counting Carbs**: Carbs are still present in vegetarian meals, so carb counting remains important. Learn to differentiate between high-glycemic index (GI) and low-GI carbs. High-

GI carbs cause blood sugar spikes, while low-GI carbs provide sustained energy.

- **Micronutrient Magic:** Certain vitamins and minerals, like vitamin B12 and iron, are more readily available from animal sources. Talk to your doctor about supplementation or incorporating fortified foods.

Meal Planning and Preparation Tips

- **Embrace Batch Cooking:** Prepare a large pot of lentil soup or a veggie chili on the weekend for easy, protein-packed lunches throughout the week.
- **Snack Savvy:** Keep healthy snacks like nuts, seeds, or veggie sticks with hummus readily available to prevent blood sugar dips.
- **Get Creative with Carbs:** Explore low-GI grains like quinoa, brown rice, and whole-wheat pasta. Pair them with non-starchy vegetables and a protein source for a balanced meal.
- **Don't Fear Fat:** Healthy fats from avocado, nuts, and olive oil can help with satiety and provide sustained energy.

Remember: They can create a personalized plan that considers your specific needs and preferences. With knowledge, planning, and a little creativity, you can enjoy a delicious vegetarian lifestyle while effectively managing your T1D.

Chapter 1: 30 Day Meal Plan

Week 1

Day 1

- Breakfast: Spinach and Feta Omelette
- Lunch: Chickpea Salad Wrap
- Dinner: Lentil Stew
- Snack: Roasted Chickpeas
- Dessert: Dark Chocolate Avocado Mousse

Day 2

- Breakfast: Greek Yogurt with Berries and Nuts
- Lunch: Quinoa and Black Bean Bowl
- Dinner: Eggplant Parmesan
- Snack: Hummus with Veggie Sticks
- Dessert: Baked Apples with Cinnamon

Day 3

- Breakfast: Avocado Toast with Cherry Tomatoes
- Lunch: Roasted Veggie Quinoa Salad
- Dinner: Tofu Stir-fry with Vegetables
- Snack: Baked Kale Chips
- Dessert: Chia Seed Pudding with Fresh Mango

Day 4

- Breakfast: Chia Seed Pudding with Almond Milk
- Lunch: Caprese Salad
- Dinner: Mushroom Risotto
- Snack: Caprese Skewers
- Dessert: Vegan Chocolate Chip Cookies

Day 5

- Breakfast: Apple Cinnamon Oatmeal
- Lunch: Cauliflower Tacos
- Dinner: Sweet Potato and Black Bean Enchiladas
- Snack: Stuffed Mini Bell Peppers
- Dessert: Berry and Yogurt Parfait

Day 6

- Breakfast: Vegetable Scramble
- Lunch: Spinach and Ricotta Stuffed Peppers
- Dinner: Cauliflower Pizza with Veggie Toppings
- Snack: Edamame with Sea Salt
- Dessert: Coconut Macaroons

Day 7

- Breakfast: Smoothie Bowl with Granola
- Lunch: Lentil and Kale Soup

- Dinner: Spaghetti Squash with Marinara Sauce
- Snack: Guacamole with Whole Grain Crackers
- Dessert: Almond Butter Brownies

Week 2

Day 8

- Breakfast: Overnight Oats with Blueberries
- Lunch: Grilled Vegetable Panini
- Dinner: Vegan Shepherd's Pie
- Snack: Veggie Spring Rolls with Peanut Sauce
- Dessert: Frozen Banana Pops

Day 9

- Breakfast: Vegan Banana Pancakes
- Lunch: Greek Salad with Tofu
- Dinner: Vegetable Paella
- Snack: Baked Zucchini Fries
- Dessert: Carrot Cake Energy Bites

Day 10

- Breakfast: Mushroom and Tomato Frittata
- Lunch: Stuffed Avocado with Chickpeas
- Dinner: Thai Green Curry with Tofu

- Snack: Spicy Roasted Almonds
- Dessert: Raspberry Sorbet

Day 11

- Breakfast: Quinoa Breakfast Bowl
- Lunch: Edamame and Cucumber Sushi Rolls
- Dinner: Stuffed Bell Peppers with Quinoa
- Snack: Cucumber and Avocado Sushi Bites
- Dessert: Date and Nut Energy Bars

Day 12

- Breakfast: Sweet Potato Hash
- Lunch: Eggplant and Zucchini Lasagna
- Dinner: Spinach and Mushroom Stuffed Shells
- Snack: Carrot and Hummus Roll-Ups
- Dessert: Lemon Chia Seed Muffins

Day 13

- Breakfast: Ricotta and Berry Toast
- Lunch: Pesto Zoodles
- Dinner: Veggie and Bean Chili
- Snack: Greek Yogurt with Cucumber and Dill
- Dessert: Apple Crumble with Oats

Day 14

- Breakfast: Tofu Breakfast Burrito
- Lunch: Falafel Wrap with Tahini Sauce
- Dinner: Grilled Portobello Mushrooms with Garlic Sauce
- Snack: Tomato Basil Bruschetta
- Dessert: Pumpkin Spice Smoothie Bowl

Week 3

Day 15

- Breakfast: Almond Flour Muffins
- Lunch: Moroccan Couscous Salad
- Dinner: Butternut Squash and Sage Risotto
- Snack: Spiced Apple Slices with Almond Butter
- Dessert: Blueberry Oat Bars

Day 16

- Breakfast: Spinach and Feta Omelette
- Lunch: Chickpea Salad Wrap
- Dinner: Lentil Stew
- Snack: Roasted Chickpeas
- Dessert: Dark Chocolate Avocado Mousse

Day 17

- Breakfast: Greek Yogurt with Berries and Nuts
- Lunch: Quinoa and Black Bean Bowl
- Dinner: Eggplant Parmesan
- Snack: Hummus with Veggie Sticks
- Dessert: Baked Apples with Cinnamon

Day 18

- Breakfast: Avocado Toast with Cherry Tomatoes
- Lunch: Roasted Veggie Quinoa Salad
- Dinner: Tofu Stir-fry with Vegetables
- Snack: Baked Kale Chips
- Dessert: Chia Seed Pudding with Fresh Mango

Day 19

- Breakfast: Chia Seed Pudding with Almond Milk
- Lunch: Caprese Salad
- Dinner: Mushroom Risotto
- Snack: Caprese Skewers
- Dessert: Vegan Chocolate Chip Cookies

Day 20

- Breakfast: Apple Cinnamon Oatmeal
- Lunch: Cauliflower Tacos

- Dinner: Sweet Potato and Black Bean Enchiladas
- Snack: Stuffed Mini Bell Peppers
- Dessert: Berry and Yogurt Parfait

Day 21

- Breakfast: Vegetable Scramble
- Lunch: Spinach and Ricotta Stuffed Peppers
- Dinner: Cauliflower Pizza with Veggie Toppings
- Snack: Edamame with Sea Salt
- Dessert: Coconut Macaroons

Week 4

Day 22

- Breakfast: Smoothie Bowl with Granola
- Lunch: Lentil and Kale Soup
- Dinner: Spaghetti Squash with Marinara Sauce
- Snack: Guacamole with Whole Grain Crackers
- Dessert: Almond Butter Brownies

Day 23

- Breakfast: Overnight Oats with Blueberries
- Lunch: Grilled Vegetable Panini
- Dinner: Vegan Shepherd's Pie

- Snack: Veggie Spring Rolls with Peanut Sauce
- Dessert: Frozen Banana Pops

Day 24

- Breakfast: Vegan Banana Pancakes
- Lunch: Greek Salad with Tofu
- Dinner: Vegetable Paella
- Snack: Baked Zucchini Fries
- Dessert: Carrot Cake Energy Bites

Day 25

- Breakfast: Mushroom and Tomato Frittata
- Lunch: Stuffed Avocado with Chickpeas
- Dinner: Thai Green Curry with Tofu
- Snack: Spicy Roasted Almonds
- Dessert: Raspberry Sorbet

Day 26

- Breakfast: Quinoa Breakfast Bowl
- Lunch: Edamame and Cucumber Sushi Rolls
- Dinner: Stuffed Bell Peppers with Quinoa
- Snack: Cucumber and Avocado Sushi Bites
- Dessert: Date and Nut Energy Bars

Day 27

- Breakfast: Sweet Potato Hash
- Lunch: Eggplant and Zucchini Lasagna
- Dinner: Spinach and Mushroom Stuffed Shells
- Snack: Carrot and Hummus Roll-Ups
- Dessert: Lemon Chia Seed Muffins

Day 28

- Breakfast: Ricotta and Berry Toast
- Lunch: Pesto Zoodles
- Dinner: Veggie and Bean Chili
- Snack: Greek Yogurt with Cucumber and Dill
- Dessert: Apple Crumble with Oats

Day 29

- Breakfast: Tofu Breakfast Burrito
- Lunch: Falafel Wrap with Tahini Sauce
- Dinner: Grilled Portobello Mushrooms with Garlic Sauce
- Snack: Tomato Basil Bruschetta
- Dessert: Pumpkin Spice Smoothie Bowl

Day 30

- Breakfast: Almond Flour Muffins
- Lunch: Moroccan Couscous Salad

- Dinner: Butternut Squash and Sage Risotto

- Snack: Spiced Apple Slices with Almond Butter

- Dessert: Blueberry Oat Bars

Chapter 2: Breakfast Recipes

This chapter provides delicious vegetarian breakfast recipes that are easy to prepare, packed with nutrients, and designed to help maintain steady blood sugar levels. Each recipe includes a balance of proteins, healthy fats, and carbohydrates, ensuring you have the energy needed to tackle your day.

Spinach and Feta Omelette

Ingredients:

- 3 large eggs
- 1 cup fresh spinach, chopped
- 1/4 cup feta cheese, crumbled
- 1 tbsp olive oil
- Salt and pepper to taste

Instructions:

1. In a bowl, beat the eggs with a pinch of salt and pepper.
2. Heat olive oil in a non-stick skillet over medium heat.
3. Add spinach and sauté until wilted.
4. Pour in the eggs and cook until they begin to set.
5. Sprinkle feta cheese on top, fold the omelette, and cook until done.

Nutrition Information (per serving):

- Calories: 320
- Protein: 20g
- Carbohydrates: 4g
- Fat: 25g
- Fiber: 1g
- Sugar: 1g
- Portion Size: 1 omelette

Greek Yogurt with Berries and Nuts

Ingredients:

- 1 cup Greek yogurt
- 1/2 cup mixed berries (blueberries, strawberries, raspberries)
- 2 tbsp mixed nuts (almonds, walnuts, pecans)
- 1 tsp honey (optional)

Instructions:

1. Scoop Greek yogurt into a bowl.
2. Top with mixed berries and nuts.
3. Drizzle with honey if desired.

Nutrition Information (per serving):

- Calories: 250

- Protein: 15g

- Carbohydrates: 20g

- Fat: 12g

- Fiber: 3g

- Sugar: 15g

- Portion Size: 1 bowl

Avocado Toast with Cherry Tomatoes

Ingredients:

- 1 slice whole grain bread

- 1/2 avocado, mashed

- 1/4 cup cherry tomatoes, halved

- Salt, pepper, and red pepper flakes to taste

Instructions:

1. Toast the bread.

2. Spread mashed avocado on the toast.

3. Top with cherry tomatoes and season with salt, pepper, and red pepper flakes.

Nutrition Information (per serving):

- Calories: 220

- Protein: 5g

- Carbohydrates: 22g

- Fat: 15g

- Fiber: 8g

- Sugar: 3g

- Portion Size: 1 slice

Chia Seed Pudding with Almond Milk

Ingredients:

- 1/4 cup chia seeds

- 1 cup unsweetened almond milk

- 1 tsp vanilla extract

- 1 tbsp maple syrup

- Fresh fruit for topping

Instructions:

1. Mix chia seeds, almond milk, vanilla extract, and maple syrup in a bowl.

2. Refrigerate for at least 4 hours or overnight.

3. Top with fresh fruit before serving.

Nutrition Information (per serving):

- Calories: 190

- Protein: 4g

- Carbohydrates: 15g

- Fat: 10g

- Fiber: 10g

- Sugar: 8g

- Portion Size: 1 bowl

Apple Cinnamon Oatmeal

Ingredients:

- 1/2 cup rolled oats

- 1 cup water or milk

- 1 apple, chopped

- 1 tsp cinnamon

- 1 tbsp chopped walnuts

- 1 tsp honey (optional)

Instructions:

1. Cook oats with water or milk according to package instructions.

2. Stir in chopped apple and cinnamon.

3. Top with walnuts and honey if desired.

Nutrition Information (per serving):

- Calories: 250

- Protein: 5g
- Carbohydrates: 45g
- Fat: 7g
- Fiber: 6g
- Sugar: 18g
- Portion Size: 1 bowl

Vegetable Scramble

Ingredients:

- 3 large eggs
- 1/4 cup bell peppers, diced
- 1/4 cup onions, diced
- 1/4 cup tomatoes, diced
- 1 tbsp olive oil
- Salt and pepper to taste

Instructions:

1. Beat eggs in a bowl with salt and pepper.
2. Heat olive oil in a skillet over medium heat.
3. Sauté bell peppers, onions, and tomatoes until soft.
4. Pour in the eggs and scramble until cooked.

Nutrition Information (per serving):

- Calories: 230
- Protein: 18g
- Carbohydrates: 6g
- Fat: 16g
- Fiber: 2g
- Sugar: 4g
- Portion Size: 1 scramble

Smoothie Bowl with Granola

Ingredients:

- 1 cup frozen mixed berries
- 1/2 banana
- 1/2 cup almond milk
- 1/4 cup granola
- Fresh fruit for topping

Instructions:

1. Blend berries, banana, and almond milk until smooth.
2. Pour into a bowl and top with granola and fresh fruit.

Nutrition Information (per serving):

- Calories: 300

- Protein: 5g
- Carbohydrates: 60g
- Fat: 8g
- Fiber: 10g
- Sugar: 30g
- Portion Size: 1 bowl

Overnight Oats with Blueberries

Ingredients:

- 1/2 cup rolled oats
- 1/2 cup unsweetened almond milk
- 1/4 cup blueberries
- 1 tbsp chia seeds
- 1 tsp maple syrup

Instructions:

1. Combine all ingredients in a jar.
2. Refrigerate overnight.
3. Stir and serve in the morning.

Nutrition Information (per serving):

- Calories: 250
- Protein: 6g

- Carbohydrates: 40g

- Fat: 8g

- Fiber: 8g

- Sugar: 10g

- Portion Size: 1 jar

Vegan Banana Pancakes

Ingredients:

- 1 cup whole wheat flour

- 1 tbsp baking powder

- 1/2 tsp salt

- 1 cup almond milk

- 1 ripe banana, mashed

- 1 tsp vanilla extract

- 1 tbsp maple syrup

Instructions:

1. Mix flour, baking powder, and salt in a bowl.

2. In another bowl, combine almond milk, mashed banana, vanilla extract, and maple syrup.

3. Pour wet ingredients into dry and mix until combined.

4. Cook pancakes on a heated griddle until bubbles form and edges are set.

Nutrition Information (per serving - 2 pancakes):

- Calories: 220
- Protein: 5g
- Carbohydrates: 40g
- Fat: 3g
- Fiber: 5g
- Sugar: 12g
- Portion Size: 2 pancakes

Mushroom and Tomato Frittata

Ingredients:

- 6 large eggs
- 1 cup mushrooms, sliced
- 1/2 cup cherry tomatoes, halved
- 1/4 cup shredded mozzarella cheese
- 1 tbsp olive oil
- Salt and pepper to taste

Instructions:

1. Preheat oven to 350°F (175°C).
2. Beat eggs in a bowl with salt and pepper.
3. Heat olive oil in an oven-safe skillet.
4. Sauté mushrooms and tomatoes until soft.

5. Pour eggs over vegetables and sprinkle with cheese.

6. Bake until eggs are set and cheese is melted.

Nutrition Information (per serving):

- Calories: 220
- Protein: 18g
- Carbohydrates: 4g
- Fat: 15g
- Fiber: 1g
- Sugar: 2g
- Portion Size: 1 slice

Quinoa Breakfast Bowl

Ingredients:

- 1/2 cup cooked quinoa
- 1/4 cup black beans
- 1/4 avocado, sliced
- 1 tbsp salsa
- 1 tbsp chopped cilantro

Instructions:

1. Place cooked quinoa in a bowl.

2. Top with black beans, avocado, salsa, and cilantro.

Nutrition Information (per serving):

- Calories: 250
- Protein: 8g
- Carbohydrates: 35g
- Fat: 9g
- Fiber: 10g
- Sugar: 2g
- Portion Size: 1 bowl

Sweet Potato Hash

Ingredients:

- 1 large sweet potato, diced
- 1/4 cup bell peppers, diced
- 1/4 cup onions, diced
- 1 tbsp olive oil
- Salt and pepper to taste

Instructions:

1. Heat olive oil in a skillet over medium heat.
2. Add sweet potato, bell peppers, and onions.
3. Cook until sweet potato is tender and golden brown, seasoning with salt and pepper.

Nutrition Information (per serving):

- Calories: 180
- Protein: 2g
- Carbohydrates: 28g
- Fat: 7g
- Fiber: 5g
- Sugar: 7g
- Portion Size: 1 cup

Ricotta and Berry Toast

Ingredients:

- 1 slice whole grain bread
- 1/4 cup ricotta cheese
- 1/4 cup mixed berries (strawberries, blueberries, raspberries)
- 1 tsp honey

Instructions:

1. Toast the bread.
2. Spread ricotta cheese on the toast.
3. Top with mixed berries and drizzle with honey.

Nutrition Information (per serving):

- Calories: 220

- Protein: 10g

- Carbohydrates: 25g

- Fat: 8g

- Fiber: 4g

- Sugar: 10g

- Portion Size: 1 slice

Tofu Breakfast Burrito

Ingredients:

- 1/2 cup crumbled firm tofu

- 1/4 cup bell peppers, diced

- 1/4 cup onions, diced

- 1 whole wheat tortilla

- 1 tbsp salsa

- 1 tbsp olive oil

- Salt and pepper to taste

Instructions:

1. Heat olive oil in a skillet over medium heat.

2. Sauté tofu, bell peppers, and onions until tofu is golden brown.

3. Season with salt and pepper.

4. Wrap mixture in a tortilla and top with salsa.

Nutrition Information (per serving):

- Calories: 250
- Protein: 12g
- Carbohydrates: 30g
- Fat: 10g
- Fiber: 6g
- Sugar: 4g
- Portion Size: 1 burrito

Almond Flour Muffins

Ingredients:

- 2 cups almond flour
- 1/2 tsp baking soda
- 1/4 tsp salt
- 3 large eggs
- 1/4 cup honey
- 1 tsp vanilla extract
- 1/4 cup unsweetened applesauce

Instructions:

1. Preheat oven to 350°F (175°C).
2. Mix almond flour, baking soda, and salt in a bowl.

3. In another bowl, whisk eggs, honey, vanilla extract, and applesauce.

4. Combine wet and dry ingredients.

5. Pour batter into muffin cups and bake for 20-25 minutes.

Nutrition Information (per serving - 1 muffin):

- Calories: 180
- Protein: 6g
- Carbohydrates: 10g
- Fat: 14g
- Fiber: 3g
- Sugar: 8g
- Portion Size: 1 muffin

Chapter 3: Lunch Recipes

These recipes focus on incorporating high-fiber, protein-rich ingredients that help maintain stable blood sugar levels. Each dish is designed to be delicious, satisfying, and easy to prepare, making your lunchtime both nutritious and enjoyable.

Chickpea Salad Wrap

Ingredients:

- 1 cup canned chickpeas, drained and rinsed
- 1/4 cup diced celery
- 1/4 cup diced red onion
- 1/4 cup diced bell pepper
- 2 tbsp vegan mayo
- 1 tsp Dijon mustard
- Salt and pepper to taste
- Whole grain wraps
- Fresh spinach leaves

Instructions:

1. Mash chickpeas in a bowl until slightly chunky.
2. Mix in celery, onion, bell pepper, mayo, and mustard.
3. Season with salt and pepper.

4. Spread the mixture onto the wrap and top with spinach leaves.

5. Roll up and serve.

Nutrition Information:

- Calories: 250
- Protein: 10g
- Carbohydrates: 35g
- Fat: 8g
- Fiber: 7g
- Sugar: 4g
- Portion size: 1 wrap

Quinoa and Black Bean Bowl

Ingredients:

- 1 cup cooked quinoa
- 1/2 cup black beans, rinsed and drained
- 1/4 cup corn kernels
- 1/4 cup diced tomatoes
- 1/4 cup diced red onion
- 1/4 cup diced avocado
- 1 tbsp olive oil
- 1 tbsp lime juice

- 1 tsp cumin

- Salt and pepper to taste

Instructions:

1. In a large bowl, combine quinoa, black beans, corn, tomatoes, red onion, and avocado.
2. Drizzle with olive oil and lime juice.
3. Sprinkle with cumin, salt, and pepper.
4. Toss to combine and serve.

Nutrition Information:

- Calories: 300

- Protein: 10g

- Carbohydrates: 45g

- Fat: 10g

- Fiber: 10g

- Sugar: 3g

- Portion size: 1 bowl

Roasted Veggie Quinoa Salad

Ingredients:

- 1 cup cooked quinoa

- 1 cup roasted vegetables (zucchini, bell peppers, carrots)

- 1/4 cup feta cheese, crumbled

- 2 tbsp olive oil

- 1 tbsp balsamic vinegar

- Salt and pepper to taste

Instructions:

1. Combine quinoa and roasted vegetables in a bowl.

2. Drizzle with olive oil and balsamic vinegar.

3. Season with salt and pepper.

4. Toss to combine and sprinkle with feta cheese.

Nutrition Information:

- Calories: 320

- Protein: 9g

- Carbohydrates: 40g

- Fat: 15g

- Fiber: 8g

- Sugar: 6g

- Portion size: 1 salad

Caprese Salad

Ingredients:

- 2 large tomatoes, sliced

- 1 ball fresh mozzarella, sliced

- Fresh basil leaves

- 2 tbsp olive oil

- 1 tbsp balsamic glaze

- Salt and pepper to taste

Instructions:

1. Arrange tomato and mozzarella slices on a plate, alternating.

2. Tuck basil leaves between slices.

3. Drizzle with olive oil and balsamic glaze.

4. Season with salt and pepper and serve.

Nutrition Information:

- Calories: 220

- Protein: 12g

- Carbohydrates: 10g

- Fat: 16g

- Fiber: 2g

- Sugar: 6g

- Portion size: 1 salad

Cauliflower Tacos

Ingredients:

- 2 cups cauliflower florets
- 1 tbsp olive oil
- 1 tsp chili powder
- 1 tsp cumin
- Salt and pepper to taste
- Corn tortillas
- Shredded lettuce
- Diced tomatoes
- Avocado slices
- Lime wedges

Instructions:

1. Preheat oven to 400°F (200°C).
2. Toss cauliflower with olive oil, chili powder, cumin, salt, and pepper.
3. Roast for 25 minutes or until tender.
4. Serve in tortillas topped with lettuce, tomatoes, avocado, and a squeeze of lime.

Nutrition Information:

- Calories: 180
- Protein: 4g

- Carbohydrates: 20g

- Fat: 9g

- Fiber: 6g

- Sugar: 4g

- Portion size: 2 tacos

Spinach and Ricotta Stuffed Peppers

Ingredients:

- 4 bell peppers, halved and seeded

- 1 cup ricotta cheese

- 1 cup spinach, chopped

- 1/4 cup grated Parmesan cheese

- 1 garlic clove, minced

- Salt and pepper to taste

Instructions:

1. Preheat oven to 375°F (190°C).

2. Mix ricotta, spinach, Parmesan, garlic, salt, and pepper in a bowl.

3. Stuff bell peppers with the mixture.

4. Place in a baking dish and bake for 30 minutes.

Nutrition Information:

- Calories: 200
- Protein: 10g
- Carbohydrates: 12g
- Fat: 12g
- Fiber: 3g
- Sugar: 6g
- Portion size: 2 halves

Lentil and Kale Soup

Ingredients:

- 1 cup lentils, rinsed
- 1 onion, diced
- 2 carrots, diced
- 2 celery stalks, diced
- 2 cups kale, chopped
- 4 cups vegetable broth
- 1 tsp thyme
- 1 bay leaf
- Salt and pepper to taste

Instructions:

1. In a large pot, sauté onion, carrots, and celery until softened.

2. Add lentils, broth, thyme, bay leaf, salt, and pepper.

3. Bring to a boil, then simmer for 30 minutes.

4. Stir in kale and cook for an additional 5 minutes.

Nutrition Information:

- Calories: 250

- Protein: 15g

- Carbohydrates: 40g

- Fat: 2g

- Fiber: 15g

- Sugar: 5g

- Portion size: 1 bowl

Grilled Vegetable Panini

Ingredients:

- 1 zucchini, sliced

- 1 bell pepper, sliced

- 1 red onion, sliced

- 1 tbsp olive oil

- Whole grain bread

- 2 tbsp hummus

- 1/4 cup spinach leaves

Instructions:

1. Toss vegetables with olive oil and grill until tender.
2. Spread hummus on bread slices.
3. Layer grilled vegetables and spinach on bread.
4. Press in a panini maker until golden and crispy.

Nutrition Information:

- Calories: 350
- Protein: 10g
- Carbohydrates: 50g
- Fat: 12g
- Fiber: 8g
- Sugar: 6g
- Portion size: 1 panini

Greek Salad with Tofu

Ingredients:

- 1 cup cubed tofu
- 1 cucumber, diced
- 2 tomatoes, diced
- 1/4 cup red onion, sliced
- 1/4 cup Kalamata olives
- 1/4 cup feta cheese

- 2 tbsp olive oil

- 1 tbsp red wine vinegar

- Salt and pepper to taste

Instructions:

1. In a large bowl, combine tofu, cucumber, tomatoes, onion, olives, and feta.
2. Drizzle with olive oil and vinegar.
3. Season with salt and pepper.
4. Toss to combine and serve.

Nutrition Information:

- Calories: 300

- Protein: 15g

- Carbohydrates: 15g

- Fat: 20g

- Fiber: 5g

- Sugar: 6g

- Portion size: 1 salad

Stuffed Avocado with Chickpeas

Ingredients:

- 2 avocados, halved and pitted

- 1 cup chickpeas, rinsed and drained
- 1/4 cup diced red onion
- 1/4 cup diced tomatoes
- 1 tbsp lime juice
- Salt and pepper to taste

Instructions:

1. In a bowl, mash chickpeas slightly.
2. Mix in onion, tomatoes, lime juice, salt, and pepper.
3. Spoon the mixture into avocado halves and serve.

Nutrition Information:

- Calories: 300
- Protein: 7g
- Carbohydrates: 25g
- Fat: 20g
- Fiber: 12g
- Sugar: 3g
- Portion size: 2 halves

Edamame and Cucumber Sushi Rolls

Ingredients:

- 1 cup cooked sushi rice

- 1/2 cup shelled edamame

- 1/2 cucumber, julienned

- Nori sheets

- Soy sauce for dipping

Instructions:

1. Spread a thin layer of sushi rice on nori sheets.

2. Arrange edamame and cucumber in the center.

3. Roll tightly and slice into pieces.

4. Serve with soy sauce.

Nutrition Information:

- Calories: 200

- Protein: 8g

- Carbohydrates: 35g

- Fat: 3g

- Fiber: 4g

- Sugar: 2g

- Portion size: 1 roll

Eggplant and Zucchini Lasagna

Ingredients:

- 1 eggplant, sliced

- 1 zucchini, sliced
- 1 cup ricotta cheese
- 1 cup marinara sauce
- 1/2 cup shredded mozzarella
- 1/4 cup grated Parmesan
- Salt and pepper to taste

Instructions:

1. Preheat oven to 375°F (190°C).
2. Layer eggplant, zucchini, ricotta, and marinara in a baking dish.
3. Top with mozzarella and Parmesan.
4. Bake for 35 minutes until bubbly and golden.

Nutrition Information:

- Calories: 320
- Protein: 15g
- Carbohydrates: 25g
- Fat: 18g
- Fiber: 6g
- Sugar: 10g
- Portion size: 1 serving

Pesto Zoodles

Ingredients:

- 2 zucchinis, spiralized
- 1/4 cup pesto sauce
- 1/4 cup cherry tomatoes, halved
- 2 tbsp pine nuts, toasted
- Salt and pepper to taste

Instructions:

1. Toss zoodles with pesto sauce in a bowl.
2. Add cherry tomatoes and pine nuts.
3. Season with salt and pepper.
4. Serve immediately.

Nutrition Information:

- Calories: 200
- Protein: 5g
- Carbohydrates: 10g
- Fat: 16g
- Fiber: 3g
- Sugar: 5g
- Portion size: 1 bowl

Falafel Wrap with Tahini Sauce

Ingredients:

- 4 falafel patties
- Whole grain wrap
- 1/4 cup shredded lettuce
- 1/4 cup diced tomatoes
- 1/4 cup cucumber slices
- 2 tbsp tahini sauce

Instructions:

1. Warm falafel patties in the oven or microwave.
2. Place falafel in the wrap.
3. Add lettuce, tomatoes, and cucumber.
4. Drizzle with tahini sauce and wrap tightly.

Nutrition Information:

- Calories: 350
- Protein: 10g
- Carbohydrates: 45g
- Fat: 15g
- Fiber: 8g
- Sugar: 4g
- Portion size: 1 wrap

Moroccan Couscous Salad

Ingredients:

- 1 cup cooked couscous
- 1/4 cup chickpeas, rinsed and drained
- 1/4 cup diced cucumber
- 1/4 cup diced bell pepper
- 1/4 cup raisins
- 2 tbsp chopped fresh mint
- 2 tbsp olive oil
- 1 tbsp lemon juice
- 1 tsp ground cumin
- Salt and pepper to taste

Instructions:

1. In a large bowl, combine couscous, chickpeas, cucumber, bell pepper, raisins, and mint.
2. Drizzle with olive oil and lemon juice.
3. Sprinkle with cumin, salt, and pepper.
4. Toss to combine and serve.

Nutrition Information:

- Calories: 280
- Protein: 8g
- Carbohydrates: 45g

- Fat: 9g
- Fiber: 6g
- Sugar: 10g
- Portion size: 1 salad

Chapter 4: Dinner Recipes

The recipes in this chapter are designed to be both nutritious and delicious, helping you maintain balanced blood sugar levels while enjoying a variety of flavors and textures. Each recipe includes detailed nutritional information to help you make informed choices.

Lentil Stew

Ingredients:

- 1 cup lentils, rinsed
- 1 onion, chopped
- 2 carrots, sliced
- 2 celery stalks, chopped
- 4 cloves garlic, minced
- 1 can diced tomatoes
- 4 cups vegetable broth
- 1 tsp cumin
- 1 tsp paprika
- Salt and pepper to taste
- 2 tbsp olive oil

Instructions:

1. Heat olive oil in a large pot over medium heat.

2. Add onion, carrots, and celery; sauté until soft.

3. Stir in garlic, cumin, and paprika; cook for 1 minute.

4. Add lentils, tomatoes, and broth; bring to a boil.

5. Reduce heat and simmer for 30-35 minutes until lentils are tender.

6. Season with salt and pepper.

Nutrition Information:

- Calories: 240
- Protein: 12g
- Carbohydrates: 38g
- Fat: 6g
- Fiber: 15g
- Sugar: 6g
- Portion size: 1 cup

Eggplant Parmesan

Ingredients:

- 2 large eggplants, sliced into rounds
- 1 cup breadcrumbs
- 1 cup grated Parmesan cheese
- 2 cups marinara sauce
- 2 cups shredded mozzarella cheese

- 2 eggs, beaten
- 1 cup flour
- 1 tsp Italian seasoning
- Olive oil spray

Instructions:

1. Preheat oven to 375°F (190°C).
2. Dip eggplant slices in flour, then egg, then breadcrumbs mixed with Parmesan and Italian seasoning.
3. Place on a baking sheet; spray with olive oil.
4. Bake for 25 minutes, flipping halfway.
5. Layer eggplant slices with marinara sauce and mozzarella in a baking dish.
6. Bake for another 20 minutes until cheese is melted and bubbly.

Nutrition Information:

- Calories: 350
- Protein: 18g
- Carbohydrates: 30g
- Fat: 18g
- Fiber: 7g
- Sugar: 8g
- Portion size: 1 cup

Tofu Stir-fry with Vegetables

Ingredients:

- 1 block firm tofu, cubed
- 2 cups mixed vegetables (bell peppers, broccoli, carrots)
- 3 tbsp soy sauce
- 1 tbsp sesame oil
- 1 tbsp olive oil
- 2 cloves garlic, minced
- 1 tsp ginger, grated
- 1 tbsp cornstarch

Instructions:

1. Toss tofu with cornstarch.
2. Heat olive oil in a pan; cook tofu until golden and crispy.
3. Remove tofu; add sesame oil, garlic, and ginger to the pan.
4. Add vegetables; stir-fry for 5-7 minutes.
5. Return tofu to the pan; add soy sauce and cook for another 2 minutes.

Nutrition Information:

- Calories: 220
- Protein: 14g
- Carbohydrates: 14g
- Fat: 12g

- Fiber: 4g

- Sugar: 4g

- Portion size: 1 cup

Mushroom Risotto

Ingredients:

- 1 cup Arborio rice

- 4 cups vegetable broth

- 1 cup mushrooms, sliced

- 1 onion, chopped

- 2 cloves garlic, minced

- 1/2 cup white wine (optional)

- 1/2 cup grated Parmesan cheese

- 2 tbsp butter

- 2 tbsp olive oil

Instructions:

1. Heat olive oil in a pan; sauté onions and garlic until soft.

2. Add mushrooms; cook until tender.

3. Stir in rice; cook for 1-2 minutes.

4. Add wine, if using; cook until absorbed.

5. Add broth, one cup at a time, stirring until absorbed before adding more.

6. Stir in butter and Parmesan before serving.

Nutrition Information:

- Calories: 350
- Protein: 10g
- Carbohydrates: 45g
- Fat: 12g
- Fiber: 3g
- Sugar: 4g
- Portion size: 1 cup

Sweet Potato and Black Bean Enchiladas

Ingredients:

- 2 large sweet potatoes, peeled and diced
- 1 can black beans, drained and rinsed
- 1 onion, chopped
- 2 cloves garlic, minced
- 1 tsp cumin
- 1 tsp chili powder
- 2 cups enchilada sauce
- 8 whole wheat tortillas
- 1 cup shredded cheese

Instructions:

1. Preheat oven to 375°F (190°C).
2. Cook sweet potatoes in a large pan until tender.
3. Add onion, garlic, beans, cumin, and chili powder; cook for 5 minutes.
4. Fill tortillas with the mixture; roll up and place in a baking dish.
5. Pour enchilada sauce over the top; sprinkle with cheese.
6. Bake for 20 minutes until bubbly.

Nutrition Information:

- Calories: 400
- Protein: 14g
- Carbohydrates: 65g
- Fat: 12g
- Fiber: 12g
- Sugar: 8g
- Portion size: 2 enchiladas

Cauliflower Pizza with Veggie Toppings

Ingredients:

- 1 head cauliflower, riced
- 1/2 cup grated Parmesan cheese

- 1/2 cup mozzarella cheese
- 1 egg, beaten
- 1 tsp Italian seasoning
- 1 cup marinara sauce
- 1 cup assorted veggies (bell peppers, mushrooms, onions)
- Olive oil spray

Instructions:

1. Preheat oven to 425°F (220°C).
2. Mix cauliflower, Parmesan, mozzarella, egg, and Italian seasoning.
3. Press mixture onto a baking sheet to form a crust.
4. Bake for 15-20 minutes until golden.
5. Top with marinara sauce and veggies; bake for another 10 minutes.

Nutrition Information:

- Calories: 280
- Protein: 15g
- Carbohydrates: 20g
- Fat: 16g
- Fiber: 6g
- Sugar: 8g
- Portion size: 2 slices

Spaghetti Squash with Marinara Sauce

Ingredients:

- 1 large spaghetti squash
- 2 cups marinara sauce
- 1 cup cherry tomatoes, halved
- 1/4 cup grated Parmesan cheese
- 2 tbsp olive oil
- Salt and pepper to taste

Instructions:

1. Preheat oven to 400°F (200°C).
2. Cut squash in half, remove seeds, and drizzle with olive oil.
3. Roast cut side down for 40 minutes.
4. Scrape out strands with a fork.
5. Heat marinara sauce; mix with spaghetti squash and tomatoes.
6. Top with Parmesan cheese.

Nutrition Information:

- Calories: 180
- Protein: 5g
- Carbohydrates: 35g
- Fat: 6g
- Fiber: 8g

- Sugar: 12g

- Portion size: 1 cup

Vegan Shepherd's Pie

Ingredients:

- 1 cup lentils, cooked

- 2 cups mixed vegetables (carrots, peas, corn)

- 4 potatoes, peeled and mashed

- 1 onion, chopped

- 2 cloves garlic, minced

- 1 cup vegetable broth

- 2 tbsp olive oil

- Salt and pepper to taste

Instructions:

1. Preheat oven to 375°F (190°C).
2. Heat olive oil in a pan; sauté onion and garlic until soft.
3. Add vegetables and broth; cook until tender.
4. Stir in lentils and season with salt and pepper.
5. Transfer to a baking dish; spread mashed potatoes on top.
6. Bake for 25 minutes until golden.

Nutrition Information:

- Calories: 300
- Protein: 10g
- Carbohydrates: 55g
- Fat: 6g
- Fiber: 10g
- Sugar: 6g
- Portion size: 1 cup

Vegetable Paella

Ingredients:

- 1 cup Arborio rice
- 1 bell pepper, chopped
- 1 cup green beans, chopped
- 1 tomato, chopped
- 1 onion, chopped
- 2 cloves garlic, minced
- 4 cups vegetable broth
- 1 tsp smoked paprika
- 1/2 tsp saffron threads
- 2 tbsp olive oil

Instructions:

1. Heat olive oil in a pan; sauté onion, garlic, and bell pepper.
2. Add rice, paprika, and saffron; cook for 2 minutes.
3. Stir in broth, green beans, and tomato.
4. Bring to a boil; reduce heat and simmer for 20 minutes until rice is tender.

Nutrition Information:

*   Calories: 280
*   Protein: 6g
*   Carbohydrates: 50g
*   Fat: 8g
*   Fiber: 6g
*   Sugar: 6g
*   Portion size: 1 cup

Thai Green Curry with Tofu

Ingredients:

*   1 block firm tofu, cubed
*   2 cups mixed vegetables (broccoli, bell peppers, zucchini)
*   2 tbsp green curry paste
*   1 can coconut milk
*   1 tbsp soy sauce

- 1 tbsp olive oil

- 1 lime, juiced

- Fresh basil leaves

Instructions:

1. Heat olive oil in a pan; cook tofu until golden.

2. Add curry paste and cook for 1 minute.

3. Stir in coconut milk, soy sauce, and vegetables.

4. Simmer for 10 minutes.

5. Add lime juice and basil before serving.

Nutrition Information:

- Calories: 350

- Protein: 14g

- Carbohydrates: 20g

- Fat: 24g

- Fiber: 6g

- Sugar: 8g

- Portion size: 1 cup

Stuffed Bell Peppers with Quinoa

Ingredients:

- 4 bell peppers, tops removed and seeds cleaned

- 1 cup cooked quinoa

- 1 can black beans, drained and rinsed

- 1 cup corn kernels

- 1 tomato, chopped

- 1 onion, chopped

- 2 cloves garlic, minced

- 1 tsp cumin

- 1 tsp chili powder

- 2 tbsp olive oil

- Salt and pepper to taste

Instructions:

1. Preheat oven to 375°F (190°C).

2. Heat olive oil in a pan; sauté onion and garlic.

3. Add quinoa, beans, corn, tomato, cumin, and chili powder; cook for 5 minutes.

4. Stuff peppers with the mixture.

5. Place in a baking dish and bake for 25 minutes.

Nutrition Information:

- Calories: 250

- Protein: 10g

- Carbohydrates: 45g

- Fat: 6g

- Fiber: 10g

- Sugar: 10g

- Portion size: 1 pepper

Spinach and Mushroom Stuffed Shells

Ingredients:

- 12 large pasta shells

- 1 cup ricotta cheese

- 1 cup spinach, chopped

- 1 cup mushrooms, chopped

- 1 cup marinara sauce

- 1/2 cup mozzarella cheese

- 2 cloves garlic, minced

- 1 tbsp olive oil

Instructions:

1. Preheat oven to 375°F (190°C).

2. Cook pasta shells according to package instructions.

3. Heat olive oil in a pan; sauté garlic, spinach, and mushrooms.

4. Mix with ricotta cheese.

5. Stuff shells with the mixture; place in a baking dish.

6. Top with marinara sauce and mozzarella; bake for 20
   minutes.

Nutrition Information:

- Calories: 300
- Protein: 15g
- Carbohydrates: 30g
- Fat: 14g
- Fiber: 4g
- Sugar: 6g
- Portion size: 3 shells

Veggie and Bean Chili

Ingredients:

- 1 can kidney beans, drained and rinsed
- 1 can black beans, drained and rinsed
- 1 can diced tomatoes
- 1 bell pepper, chopped
- 1 onion, chopped
- 2 cloves garlic, minced
- 2 cups vegetable broth
- 1 tsp cumin
- 1 tsp chili powder

- 2 tbsp olive oil

Instructions:

1. Heat olive oil in a pot; sauté onion, garlic, and bell pepper.
2. Add beans, tomatoes, broth, cumin, and chili powder.
3. Bring to a boil; reduce heat and simmer for 30 minutes.

Nutrition Information:

- Calories: 250
- Protein: 12g
- Carbohydrates: 40g
- Fat: 6g
- Fiber: 10g
- Sugar: 6g
- Portion size: 1 cup

Grilled Portobello Mushrooms with Garlic Sauce

Ingredients:

- 4 large portobello mushrooms
- 2 tbsp olive oil
- 4 cloves garlic, minced
- 1 tbsp balsamic vinegar

- Salt and pepper to taste
- Fresh parsley for garnish

Instructions:

1. Preheat grill to medium-high heat.
2. Brush mushrooms with olive oil and balsamic vinegar.
3. Grill for 5-7 minutes per side.
4. Mix garlic with a little olive oil; drizzle over mushrooms.
5. Garnish with parsley.

Nutrition Information:

- Calories: 150
- Protein: 4g
- Carbohydrates: 12g
- Fat: 10g
- Fiber: 3g
- Sugar: 4g
- Portion size: 1 mushroom

Butternut Squash and Sage Risotto

Ingredients:

- 1 cup Arborio rice
- 1 small butternut squash, peeled and diced

- 1 onion, chopped

- 4 cups vegetable broth

- 1/4 cup white wine (optional)

- 1/4 cup grated Parmesan cheese

- 2 tbsp butter

- 2 tbsp olive oil

- Fresh sage leaves

Instructions:

1. Heat olive oil in a pan; sauté onion and butternut squash until tender.

2. Add rice; cook for 1-2 minutes.

3. Stir in wine, if using; cook until absorbed.

4. Add broth, one cup at a time, stirring until absorbed before adding more.

5. Stir in butter, Parmesan, and sage before serving.

Nutrition Information:

- Calories: 320

- Protein: 8g

- Carbohydrates: 55g

- Fat: 10g

- Fiber: 5g

- Sugar: 8g

- Portion size: 1 cup

Chapter 5: Snacks and Appetizers

In this chapter, you'll discover an array of nutritious and delicious snacks and appetizers that are perfect for any occasion. From crunchy roasted chickpeas to refreshing cucumber and avocado sushi bites, these recipes are designed to satisfy your cravings while providing wholesome ingredients.

Roasted Chickpeas

Ingredients:

- 1 can chickpeas, drained and rinsed
- 1 tbsp olive oil
- 1 tsp paprika
- 1/2 tsp garlic powder
- Salt and pepper to taste

Instructions:

1. Preheat oven to 400°F (200°C).
2. Toss chickpeas with olive oil, paprika, garlic powder, salt, and pepper.
3. Spread on a baking sheet and roast for 25-30 minutes, stirring occasionally, until crispy.

Nutrition Information (per serving):

- Calories: 120
- Protein: 5g
- Carbohydrates: 18g
- Fat: 3g
- Fiber: 6g
- Sugar: 1g
- Portion Size: 1/2 cup

Hummus with Veggie Sticks

Ingredients:

- 1 can chickpeas, drained and rinsed
- 1/4 cup tahini
- 2 tbsp olive oil
- 2 tbsp lemon juice
- 2 cloves garlic
- Salt to taste
- Assorted veggie sticks (carrots, celery, bell peppers)

Instructions:

1. Blend chickpeas, tahini, olive oil, lemon juice, garlic, and salt until smooth.
2. Serve with assorted veggie sticks.

Nutrition Information (per serving):

- Calories: 150
- Protein: 4g
- Carbohydrates: 15g
- Fat: 9g
- Fiber: 5g
- Sugar: 2g
- Portion Size: 1/4 cup hummus with veggie sticks

Baked Kale Chips

Ingredients:

- 1 bunch kale, washed and torn into pieces
- 1 tbsp olive oil
- Salt to taste

Instructions:

1. Preheat oven to 350°F (175°C).
2. Toss kale with olive oil and salt.
3. Spread on a baking sheet and bake for 10-15 minutes until crispy.

Nutrition Information (per serving):

- Calories: 60

- Protein: 3g
- Carbohydrates: 7g
- Fat: 2g
- Fiber: 2g
- Sugar: 1g
- Portion Size: 1 cup

Caprese Skewers

Ingredients:

- Cherry tomatoes
- Fresh mozzarella balls
- Fresh basil leaves
- Balsamic glaze

Instructions:

1. Thread cherry tomatoes, mozzarella, and basil onto skewers.
2. Drizzle with balsamic glaze.

Nutrition Information (per serving):

- Calories: 80
- Protein: 4g
- Carbohydrates: 4g
- Fat: 6g

- Fiber: 1g

- Sugar: 3g

- Portion Size: 3 skewers

Stuffed Mini Bell Peppers

Ingredients:

- Mini bell peppers

- 1 cup cream cheese

- 1/4 cup chopped chives

- 1/4 cup diced tomatoes

- Salt and pepper to taste

Instructions:

1. Cut tops off mini bell peppers and remove seeds.

2. Mix cream cheese, chives, tomatoes, salt, and pepper.

3. Stuff peppers with cream cheese mixture.

Nutrition Information (per serving):

- Calories: 90

- Protein: 2g

- Carbohydrates: 4g

- Fat: 7g

- Fiber: 1g

- Sugar: 3g
- Portion Size: 4 peppers

Edamame with Sea Salt

Ingredients:

- 2 cups edamame (in pods)
- Sea salt

Instructions:

1. Boil edamame for 5 minutes.
2. Drain and sprinkle with sea salt.

Nutrition Information (per serving):

- Calories: 100
- Protein: 8g
- Carbohydrates: 9g
- Fat: 4g
- Fiber: 4g
- Sugar: 1g
- Portion Size: 1 cup

Guacamole with Whole Grain Crackers

Ingredients:

- 2 avocados, mashed
- 1/4 cup diced red onion
- 1 tomato, diced
- 1 tbsp lime juice
- Salt and pepper to taste
- Whole grain crackers

Instructions:

1. Mix avocados, red onion, tomato, lime juice, salt, and pepper.
2. Serve with whole grain crackers.

Nutrition Information (per serving):

- Calories: 150
- Protein: 2g
- Carbohydrates: 15g
- Fat: 10g
- Fiber: 6g
- Sugar: 1g
- Portion Size: 1/4 cup guacamole with crackers

Veggie Spring Rolls with Peanut Sauce

Ingredients:

- Rice paper wrappers
- 1 cup shredded carrots
- 1 cup shredded cabbage
- 1 cucumber, julienned
- 1/4 cup cilantro
- 1/4 cup mint leaves
- Peanut sauce

Instructions:

1. Soak rice paper wrappers in water until soft.
2. Fill with carrots, cabbage, cucumber, cilantro, and mint.
3. Roll tightly and serve with peanut sauce.

Nutrition Information (per serving):

- Calories: 120
- Protein: 3g
- Carbohydrates: 20g
- Fat: 3g
- Fiber: 3g
- Sugar: 4g
- Portion Size: 2 rolls

Baked Zucchini Fries

Ingredients:

- 2 zucchinis, cut into fries
- 1/2 cup breadcrumbs
- 1/4 cup grated Parmesan
- 1 egg, beaten
- Salt and pepper to taste

Instructions:

1. Preheat oven to 425°F (220°C).
2. Dip zucchini in egg, then coat with breadcrumbs and Parmesan.
3. Bake for 20-25 minutes until crispy.

Nutrition Information (per serving):

- Calories: 110
- Protein: 5g
- Carbohydrates: 12g
- Fat: 5g
- Fiber: 2g
- Sugar: 2g
- Portion Size: 1 cup

Spicy Roasted Almonds

Ingredients:

- 1 cup almonds
- 1 tbsp olive oil
- 1 tsp chili powder
- 1/2 tsp cumin
- Salt to taste

Instructions:

1. Preheat oven to 350°F (175°C).
2. Toss almonds with olive oil, chili powder, cumin, and salt.
3. Spread on a baking sheet and roast for 15 minutes.

Nutrition Information (per serving):

- Calories: 170
- Protein: 6g
- Carbohydrates: 6g
- Fat: 15g
- Fiber: 4g
- Sugar: 1g
- Portion Size: 1/4 cup

Cucumber and Avocado Sushi Bites

Ingredients:

- 1 cucumber, sliced
- 1 avocado, sliced
- Soy sauce for dipping

Instructions:

1. Top cucumber slices with avocado.
2. Serve with soy sauce for dipping.

Nutrition Information (per serving):

- Calories: 80
- Protein: 1g
- Carbohydrates: 5g
- Fat: 6g
- Fiber: 3g
- Sugar: 1g
- Portion Size: 8 pieces

Carrot and Hummus Roll-Ups

Ingredients:

- 2 large carrots, peeled into strips
- 1/2 cup hummus

- 1/4 cup chopped parsley

Instructions:

1. Spread hummus on carrot strips.
2. Sprinkle with parsley and roll up.

Nutrition Information (per serving):

- Calories: 60
- Protein: 2g
- Carbohydrates: 10g
- Fat: 2g
- Fiber: 3g
- Sugar: 4g
- Portion Size: 6 roll-ups

Greek Yogurt with Cucumber and Dill

Ingredients:

- 1 cup Greek yogurt
- 1/2 cucumber, diced
- 1 tbsp fresh dill, chopped
- Salt and pepper to taste

Instructions:

1. Mix Greek yogurt, cucumber, dill, salt, and pepper.
2. Serve chilled.

Nutrition Information (per serving):

- Calories: 100
- Protein: 10g
- Carbohydrates: 5g
- Fat: 4g
- Fiber: 1g
- Sugar: 4g
- Portion Size: 1 cup

Tomato Basil Bruschetta

Ingredients:

- 1 baguette, sliced
- 2 tomatoes, diced
- 1/4 cup fresh basil, chopped
- 2 tbsp olive oil
- 1 clove garlic, minced
- Salt and pepper to taste

Instructions:

1. Preheat oven to 375°F (190°C).
2. Toast baguette slices for 5-7 minutes.
3. Mix tomatoes, basil, olive oil, garlic, salt, and pepper.
4. Top toasted baguette with tomato mixture.

Nutrition Information (per serving):

- Calories: 90
- Protein: 2g
- Carbohydrates: 10g
- Fat: 4g
- Fiber: 1g
- Sugar: 2g
- Portion Size: 3 pieces

Spiced Apple Slices with Almond Butter

Ingredients:

- 1 apple, sliced
- 2 tbsp almond butter
- 1/2 tsp cinnamon

Instructions:

1. Spread almond butter on apple slices.

2. Sprinkle with cinnamon.

Nutrition Information (per serving):

- Calories: 150
- Protein: 3g
- Carbohydrates: 20g
- Fat: 7g
- Fiber: 5g
- Sugar: 15g
- Portion Size: 1 apple

Chapter 6: Desserts

In this chapter, we delve into a delightful array of 15 desserts that are not only delicious but also nutritious. From rich, chocolatey treats to refreshing fruit-based delights, these recipes cater to a variety of tastes and dietary preferences.

Dark Chocolate Avocado Mousse

Ingredients:

- 2 ripe avocados
- 1/2 cup unsweetened cocoa powder
- 1/4 cup maple syrup
- 1/4 cup almond milk
- 1 tsp vanilla extract
- Pinch of salt

Instructions:

1. Scoop out the avocado flesh and blend until smooth.
2. Add cocoa powder, maple syrup, almond milk, vanilla extract, and salt.
3. Blend until creamy and well combined.
4. Chill in the refrigerator for 30 minutes before serving.

Nutrition Information (per serving):

- Calories: 250
- Protein: 3g
- Carbohydrates: 24g
- Fat: 18g
- Fiber: 10g
- Sugar: 10g
- Portion Size: 1/2 cup

Baked Apples with Cinnamon

Ingredients:

- 4 apples
- 1/4 cup maple syrup
- 1 tsp ground cinnamon
- 1/4 cup chopped nuts (optional)

Instructions:

1. Preheat oven to 350°F (175°C).
2. Core the apples and place them in a baking dish.
3. Drizzle maple syrup over the apples and sprinkle with cinnamon.
4. Add chopped nuts if desired.
5. Bake for 25-30 minutes, until apples are tender.

Nutrition Information (per serving):

- Calories: 150
- Protein: 1g
- Carbohydrates: 40g
- Fat: 2g
- Fiber: 6g
- Sugar: 30g
- Portion Size: 1 apple

Chia Seed Pudding with Fresh Mango

Ingredients:

- 1/4 cup chia seeds
- 1 cup almond milk
- 1 tbsp maple syrup
- 1 fresh mango, diced

Instructions:

1. Combine chia seeds, almond milk, and maple syrup in a bowl.
2. Stir well and refrigerate for at least 4 hours or overnight.
3. Serve topped with fresh mango.

Nutrition Information (per serving):

- Calories: 200
- Protein: 4g
- Carbohydrates: 35g
- Fat: 7g
- Fiber: 10g
- Sugar: 20g
- Portion Size: 1/2 cup

Vegan Chocolate Chip Cookies

Ingredients:

- 1 cup almond flour
- 1/4 cup coconut oil, melted
- 1/4 cup maple syrup
- 1 tsp vanilla extract
- 1/2 cup vegan chocolate chips

Instructions:

1. Preheat oven to 350°F (175°C).
2. Mix almond flour, coconut oil, maple syrup, and vanilla extract until combined.
3. Fold in chocolate chips.
4. Scoop dough onto a baking sheet and flatten slightly.

5. Bake for 10-12 minutes until golden brown.

Nutrition Information (per serving):

- Calories: 120
- Protein: 2g
- Carbohydrates: 12g
- Fat: 8g
- Fiber: 2g
- Sugar: 7g
- Portion Size: 1 cookie

Berry and Yogurt Parfait

Ingredients:

- 1 cup Greek yogurt
- 1/2 cup mixed berries
- 1 tbsp honey
- 1/4 cup granola

Instructions:

1. Layer Greek yogurt, mixed berries, and honey in a glass.
2. Top with granola.
3. Serve immediately.

Nutrition Information (per serving):

- Calories: 200
- Protein: 10g
- Carbohydrates: 30g
- Fat: 5g
- Fiber: 3g
- Sugar: 18g
- Portion Size: 1 cup

Coconut Macaroons

Ingredients:

- 2 cups shredded coconut
- 1/2 cup sweetened condensed milk
- 1 tsp vanilla extract

Instructions:

1. Preheat oven to 325°F (165°C).
2. Mix shredded coconut, sweetened condensed milk, and vanilla extract.
3. Scoop mixture onto a baking sheet.
4. Bake for 15-20 minutes until golden brown.

Nutrition Information (per serving):

- Calories: 140
- Protein: 2g
- Carbohydrates: 16g
- Fat: 8g
- Fiber: 2g
- Sugar: 12g
- Portion Size: 1 macaroon

Almond Butter Brownies

Ingredients:

- 1 cup almond butter
- 1/2 cup cocoa powder
- 1/2 cup maple syrup
- 2 eggs
- 1 tsp vanilla extract
- 1/4 tsp salt

Instructions:

1. Preheat oven to 350°F (175°C).
2. Mix all ingredients in a bowl until smooth.
3. Pour batter into a greased baking pan.
4. Bake for 20-25 minutes until set.

Nutrition Information (per serving):

- Calories: 200
- Protein: 5g
- Carbohydrates: 18g
- Fat: 12g
- Fiber: 4g
- Sugar: 10g
- Portion Size: 1 brownie

Frozen Banana Pops

Ingredients:

- 4 bananas
- 1/2 cup dark chocolate chips, melted
- 1/4 cup crushed nuts or sprinkles

Instructions:

1. Peel bananas and cut them in half.
2. Insert a popsicle stick into each banana half.
3. Dip bananas in melted chocolate and sprinkle with nuts or sprinkles.
4. Freeze for at least 2 hours before serving.

Nutrition Information (per serving):

- Calories: 180
- Protein: 2g
- Carbohydrates: 34g
- Fat: 7g
- Fiber: 3g
- Sugar: 20g
- Portion Size: 1 pop

Carrot Cake Energy Bites

Ingredients:

- 1 cup grated carrots
- 1 cup rolled oats
- 1/2 cup almond butter
- 1/4 cup honey
- 1 tsp cinnamon

Instructions:

1. Combine all ingredients in a bowl.
2. Roll mixture into balls.
3. Refrigerate for at least 1 hour before serving.

Nutrition Information (per serving):

- Calories: 100
- Protein: 3g
- Carbohydrates: 15g
- Fat: 5g
- Fiber: 2g
- Sugar: 8g
- Portion Size: 2 bites

Raspberry Sorbet

Ingredients:

- 4 cups raspberries
- 1/2 cup sugar
- 1/2 cup water
- 1 tbsp lemon juice

Instructions:

1. Blend raspberries, sugar, water, and lemon juice until smooth.
2. Strain mixture to remove seeds.
3. Freeze for 4 hours, stirring every hour.

Nutrition Information (per serving):

- Calories: 120
- Protein: 1g
- Carbohydrates: 30g
- Fat: 0g
- Fiber: 6g
- Sugar: 24g
- Portion Size: 1/2 cup

Date and Nut Energy Bars

Ingredients:

- 1 cup dates
- 1/2 cup almonds
- 1/2 cup walnuts
- 1/4 cup shredded coconut
- 1 tbsp chia seeds

Instructions:

1. Blend dates, almonds, and walnuts until crumbly.
2. Add shredded coconut and chia seeds, and blend until combined.
3. Press mixture into a pan and refrigerate for 2 hours.
4. Cut into bars.

Nutrition Information (per serving):

- Calories: 180
- Protein: 4g
- Carbohydrates: 22g
- Fat: 9g
- Fiber: 4g
- Sugar: 16g
- Portion Size: 1 bar

Lemon Chia Seed Muffins

Ingredients:

- 2 cups almond flour
- 1/4 cup chia seeds
- 1/4 cup honey
- 1/4 cup lemon juice
- 2 eggs
- 1 tsp baking powder

Instructions:

1. Preheat oven to 350°F (175°C).
2. Mix all ingredients until well combined.
3. Scoop batter into muffin cups.
4. Bake for 20-25 minutes until a toothpick comes out clean.

Nutrition Information (per serving):

- Calories: 150
- Protein: 4g
- Carbohydrates: 18g
- Fat: 8g
- Fiber: 4g
- Sugar: 8g
- Portion Size: 1 muffin

Apple Crumble with Oats

Ingredients:

- 4 apples, sliced
- 1/2 cup rolled oats
- 1/4 cup almond flour
- 1/4 cup coconut oil, melted
- 2 tbsp maple syrup
- 1 tsp cinnamon

Instructions:

1. Preheat oven to 350°F (175°C).
2. Place sliced apples in a baking dish.
3. Mix oats, almond flour, coconut oil, maple syrup, and cinnamon.

4. Sprinkle mixture over apples.

5. Bake for 30-35 minutes until apples are tender and topping
    is golden.

Nutrition Information (per serving):

- Calories: 200

- Protein: 2g

- Carbohydrates: 32g

- Fat: 8g

- Fiber: 5g

- Sugar: 18g

- Portion Size: 1/2 cup

Pumpkin Spice Smoothie Bowl

Ingredients:

- 1 cup pumpkin puree

- 1 banana

- 1/2 cup almond milk

- 1 tbsp maple syrup

- 1 tsp pumpkin spice

- Toppings: granola, nuts, seeds

Instructions:

1. Blend pumpkin puree, banana, almond milk, maple syrup, and pumpkin spice until smooth.
2. Pour into a bowl and add toppings.

Nutrition Information (per serving):

- Calories: 180
- Protein: 3g
- Carbohydrates: 35g
- Fat: 4g
- Fiber: 6g
- Sugar: 18g
- Portion Size: 1 bowl

Blueberry Oat Bars

Ingredients:

- 1 cup rolled oats
- 1/2 cup almond flour
- 1/4 cup coconut oil, melted
- 1/4 cup honey
- 1 cup blueberries

Instructions:

1. Preheat oven to 350°F (175°C).
2. Mix oats, almond flour, coconut oil, and honey.
3. Press half the mixture into a baking pan.
4. Spread blueberries over the base.
5. Sprinkle remaining oat mixture on top.
6. Bake for 25-30 minutes until golden brown.

Nutrition Information (per serving):

- Calories: 150
- Protein: 2g
- Carbohydrates: 22g
- Fat: 7g
- Fiber: 3g
- Sugar: 12g
- Portion Size: 1 bar

Chapter 7: Smoothies

They can be enjoyed as a quick breakfast, a post-workout snack, or a refreshing treat any time of the day. In this chapter, you'll find unique smoothie recipes that cater to different taste preferences and nutritional needs.

Green Detox Smoothie

Ingredients:

- 1 cup spinach
- 1/2 cucumber
- 1 green apple, cored and chopped
- 1/2 lemon, juiced
- 1/2 inch ginger, peeled and grated
- 1 cup water
- Ice cubes (optional)

Instructions:

1. Place all ingredients in a blender.
2. Blend until smooth.
3. Add ice cubes if desired and blend again.

Nutrition Information:

- Calories: 90
- Protein: 2g
- Carbohydrates: 21g
- Fat: 0.5g
- Fiber: 4g
- Sugar: 12g
- Portion size: 1 glass (about 12 oz)

Strawberry Banana Smoothie

Ingredients:

- 1 banana
- 1 cup strawberries, hulled
- 1/2 cup Greek yogurt
- 1/2 cup almond milk
- 1 tablespoon honey (optional)

Instructions:

1. Combine all ingredients in a blender.
2. Blend until smooth.

Nutrition Information:

- Calories: 200

- Protein: 6g

- Carbohydrates: 39g

- Fat: 3g

- Fiber: 4g

- Sugar: 26g

- Portion size: 1 glass (about 12 oz)

Mango and Pineapple Smoothie

Ingredients:

- 1 cup mango, peeled and chopped

- 1 cup pineapple chunks

- 1/2 cup coconut water

- 1/2 cup orange juice

Instructions:

1. Add all ingredients to a blender.

2. Blend until smooth.

Nutrition Information:

- Calories: 160

- Protein: 1g

- Carbohydrates: 40g

- Fat: 0.5g

- Fiber: 4g

- Sugar: 32g

- Portion size: 1 glass (about 12 oz)

Blueberry Almond Smoothie

Ingredients:

- 1 cup blueberries

- 1/2 cup almond milk

- 1/2 banana

- 1 tablespoon almond butter

- 1 teaspoon chia seeds

Instructions:

1. Blend all ingredients together until smooth.

Nutrition Information:

- Calories: 220

- Protein: 5g

- Carbohydrates: 32g

- Fat: 10g

- Fiber: 6g

- Sugar: 15g

- Portion size: 1 glass (about 12 oz)

Chocolate Protein Smoothie

Ingredients:

- 1 banana
- 1 scoop chocolate protein powder
- 1 tablespoon peanut butter
- 1 cup almond milk
- Ice cubes (optional)

Instructions:

1. Place all ingredients in a blender.
2. Blend until smooth.

Nutrition Information:

- Calories: 300
- Protein: 20g
- Carbohydrates: 30g
- Fat: 12g
- Fiber: 5g
- Sugar: 15g
- Portion size: 1 glass (about 12 oz)

Tropical Green Smoothie

Ingredients:

- 1 cup spinach
- 1/2 cup mango
- 1/2 cup pineapple
- 1/2 banana
- 1 cup coconut water

Instructions:

1. Combine all ingredients in a blender.
2. Blend until smooth.

Nutrition Information:

- Calories: 150
- Protein: 2g
- Carbohydrates: 38g
- Fat: 0.5g
- Fiber: 4g
- Sugar: 30g
- Portion size: 1 glass (about 12 oz)

Raspberry Peach Smoothie

Ingredients:

- 1 cup raspberries
- 1 peach, pitted and chopped
- 1/2 cup Greek yogurt
- 1/2 cup orange juice

Instructions:

1. Blend all ingredients until smooth.

Nutrition Information:

- Calories: 180
- Protein: 6g
- Carbohydrates: 35g
- Fat: 2g
- Fiber: 7g
- Sugar: 26g
- Portion size: 1 glass (about 12 oz)

Spinach and Apple Smoothie

Ingredients:

- 1 cup spinach
- 1 green apple, cored and chopped

- 1/2 banana
- 1 cup water
- 1 teaspoon honey (optional)

Instructions:

1. Blend all ingredients together until smooth.

Nutrition Information:

- Calories: 120
- Protein: 2g
- Carbohydrates: 30g
- Fat: 0.5g
- Fiber: 5g
- Sugar: 18g
- Portion size: 1 glass (about 12 oz)

Beet and Berry Smoothie

Ingredients:

- 1 small beet, peeled and chopped
- 1/2 cup strawberries
- 1/2 cup blueberries
- 1/2 cup Greek yogurt
- 1 cup water

Instructions:

1. Place all ingredients in a blender.
2. Blend until smooth.

Nutrition Information:

- Calories: 150
- Protein: 6g
- Carbohydrates: 28g
- Fat: 1g
- Fiber: 5g
- Sugar: 20g
- Portion size: 1 glass (about 12 oz)

Avocado and Kale Smoothie

Ingredients:

- 1/2 avocado
- 1 cup kale
- 1/2 banana
- 1 cup almond milk

Instructions:

1. Blend all ingredients until smooth.

Nutrition Information:

- Calories: 220
- Protein: 3g
- Carbohydrates: 20g
- Fat: 15g
- Fiber: 7g
- Sugar: 7g
- Portion size: 1 glass (about 12 oz)

Orange Creamsicle Smoothie

Ingredients:

- 1 orange, peeled and segmented
- 1/2 cup Greek yogurt
- 1/2 cup orange juice
- 1 teaspoon vanilla extract
- Ice cubes (optional)

Instructions:

1. Combine all ingredients in a blender.
2. Blend until smooth.

Nutrition Information:

- Calories: 140

- Protein: 5g

- Carbohydrates: 28g

- Fat: 1g

- Fiber: 2g

- Sugar: 24g

- Portion size: 1 glass (about 12 oz)

Carrot Ginger Smoothie

Ingredients:

- 1 cup carrots, chopped

- 1/2 inch ginger, peeled and grated

- 1/2 banana

- 1 cup orange juice

Instructions:

1. Blend all ingredients together until smooth.

Nutrition Information:

- Calories: 130

- Protein: 2g

- Carbohydrates: 31g

- Fat: 0.5g

- Fiber: 4g

- Sugar: 20g

- Portion size: 1 glass (about 12 oz)

Pineapple Coconut Smoothie

Ingredients:

- 1 cup pineapple chunks

- 1/2 cup coconut milk

- 1/2 banana

- 1 tablespoon shredded coconut

Instructions:

1. Place all ingredients in a blender.

2. Blend until smooth.

Nutrition Information:

- Calories: 210

- Protein: 2g

- Carbohydrates: 30g

- Fat: 10g

- Fiber: 4g

- Sugar: 20g

- Portion size: 1 glass (about 12 oz)

Mixed Berry Smoothie

Ingredients:

- 1/2 cup strawberries
- 1/2 cup blueberries
- 1/2 cup raspberries
- 1/2 cup Greek yogurt
- 1 cup almond milk

Instructions:

1. Blend all ingredients until smooth.

Nutrition Information:

- Calories: 180
- Protein: 6g
- Carbohydrates: 30g
- Fat: 5g
- Fiber: 6g
- Sugar: 20g
- Portion size: 1 glass (about 12 oz)

Watermelon Mint Smoothie

Ingredients:

- 1 cup watermelon, chopped

- 1/2 cucumber

- 1/4 cup mint leaves

- 1/2 lime, juiced

- Ice cubes (optional)

Instructions:

1. Combine all ingredients in a blender.

2. Blend until smooth.

Nutrition Information:

- Calories: 80

- Protein: 1g

- Carbohydrates: 20g

- Fat: 0.5g

- Fiber: 1g

- Sugar: 17g

- Portion size: 1 glass (about 12 oz)

CONCLUSION

Congratulations on completing the journey through our "Type 1 Diabetic Vegetarian Cookbook"! This book is not just a collection of recipes; it's a testament to the power of delicious, nutritious, and diabetes-friendly vegetarian meals. As you've explored the chapters, you've discovered a wealth of flavors, textures, and ingredients that nourish both body and soul.

In these pages, we've woven together the intricate tapestry of a balanced diet tailored specifically for individuals managing type 1 diabetes. From hearty breakfasts to satisfying dinners, from wholesome snacks to indulgent desserts, each recipe has been meticulously crafted to strike the perfect balance between taste and health.

But this book is more than just a guide to cooking; it's a companion on your journey to better health. As you've navigated through the chapters, you've gained valuable insights into the intricate relationship between food and diabetes management. You've learned how to make informed choices, adapt recipes to suit your needs, and embrace the vibrant world of vegetarian cuisine.

As you close the book, remember that this is just the beginning of your culinary adventure. Armed with the knowledge and recipes within these pages, you now have the tools to embark on a lifelong journey of delicious and nutritious eating. Whether you're cooking for yourself, your family, or friends, may each meal be a celebration of health, happiness, and flavor.

Thank you for joining us on this flavorful journey. Here's to many more delicious meals and joyful moments in the kitchen. Bon appétit and happy cooking!

www.ingramcontent.com/pod-product-compliance
Lightning Source LLC
Chambersburg PA
CBHW061655250726
48659CB00004B/1511